33 Ways to Get Rid of Parasites

How To Cleanse Parasites For People and Pets With All-Natural Methods

Stephen Tvedten

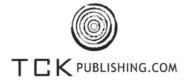

TCK PUBLISHING.COM

ISBN: **978-1-63161-101-8**

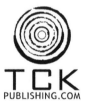

Published by TCK Publishing
www.TCKpublishing.com

Get discounts and special deals on our best-selling books at
www.TCKpublishing.com/bookdeals

Disclaimer

The information presented in this book is for educational and informational purposes only. It is not intended to be a substitute for proper diagnosis and treatment by a licensed professional. If you have any questions about whether the information and advice presented in this book is suitable for you, please check with your trusted physician or health care provider. It is your responsibility to discern if information is useful for your health and to use this guide appropriately.

The information provided herein by the author is provided "as is" and you read and use this information at your own risk. The publisher and author disclaim any liabilities for any loss of profit or commercial or personal damages resulting from the use of the information contained in this book.

Table of Contents

Why You Should Read This Book

*"In fact, parasites have killed more humans
than all the wars in history."*
—National Geographic's *The Body Snatchers*

What is a parasite? A parasite is an organism that cannot live independently without a host like you. Parasites live by taking nourishment from a host, such as humans or other animals. Their invasions are very common in humans—far more common than most people think—especially in children and the elderly, across all genders, races, and nationalities. The most common of these parasites are intestinal worms, which are a problem in all countries around the world, but especially so in less-developed countries.

How do you get parasites like worms? Usually it's because of poor food hygiene. You can ingest tiny eggs that are unnoticeable to the human eye in contaminated food or water. These worms live in your gastrointestinal tract, where they depend on the food you eat in order to live. Once parasites enter your body, they can produce toxic waste that may attack your immune system and cause destruction to your cells faster than your cells can reproduce, which can cause many diseases, symptoms, and distress.

There are several ways parasites can enter your body: through contaminated water or food (particularly meat), mosquitoes, sexual contact, the nose or mouth after touching an infected animal, or by direct contact with an open wound from a contaminated surface. Generally, a healthy person's body should kill parasites effectively and prevent them from causing any long-term health problems.

But when your immune system is weak or your digestive system is functioning poorly, parasites, like intestinal worms, can become a big problem. Parasites can create a variety of sometimes baffling symptoms, and many medical doctors don't always know how to properly diagnose such symptoms. The difficulty in diagnosing intestinal parasites is that the symptoms often mimic other health problems. Experts in human parasites have said that the infestation of parasites often goes unnoticed and therefore undiagnosed and untreated!

A conservative estimate is that 85% of people in North America and Europe are currently infected with parasites. Some authorities feel that this figure may be as high as 95%. There are more kinds of human parasites than there are people on the earth! That's over seven billion (of which 75,000 to 300,000 species are parasitic worms, with the other major parasites being protozoa, fungi, bacteria, and viruses).

Nearly everyone has parasites of one kind or another. We get them from flies, our food, the air we breathe, unclean water, each other, and even our pets. Most parasites are microscopic and very difficult to detect. You can become infected simply by inhaling dust that contains parasitic eggs or cysts, and you won't even know it unless symptoms develop and are properly diagnosed by a medical professional.

Do you eat fresh fruit, salads, raw vegetables, or sushi?

Do you eat out at restaurants?

Do you ever put your fingers in your mouth?

Have you ever been bitten by an insect? Do you ever walk around barefoot?

If so, you probably have parasites living in you! Parasites can sap your strength and energy, live off the nutrients from your food and the tissues of your body, and poison your body with the toxins they secrete.

Parasites will weaken your immune system, and they can cause many physical diseases most doctors can't identify. If you or someone you know has ongoing medical problems for which Western medicine has no answers, there's a good chance parasites are involved.

Parasites infect billions of people around the world. The vast majority of people infected with parasites do not even realize it, either because they have no symptoms, or because they confuse their symptoms with some other illness.

Parasites have been living inside us for as long as we humans have been around. About half the world's population (over three billion people) are infected with at least one of the three worms that form what Columbia University parasitologist Dickson Despommier calls the "unholy trinity": large roundworms, hookworms, and whipworms.

Most of those afflicted live in developing countries, where there is not enough clean drinking water or effective sanitation to keep infected feces from contaminating food and water, and where human excrement is used to fertilize crops.

The most prolific parasitic worm in the U.S. and European Union is the pinworm, or "threadworm" (Enterobius vermicularis), which you're most likely to encounter during childhood. It's a mystery to me why every generation prior to modern times made de-worming and internal parasite cleansing a regular part of their lives and traditions, but our generation has largely chosen to ignore parasite infestations. When's the last time someone in your neighborhood had a de-worming party? Such a social gathering sounds crazy, but it was a commonplace practice for all of human history before the modern era.

These unwanted, invisible invaders live in and feed off of you, depriving you of vitamins, nutrients, and amino acids, while altering natural pH levels, decreasing energy levels, and wreaking havoc on various organ systems. It is therefore crucial that through dietary choices and herbal supplementation (and medication when necessary) you keep your body equipped to remove these harmful invaders and prevent them from coming back.

Several parasites have emerged as significant causes of foodborne and waterborne illness. These organisms live and reproduce within the tissues and organs of infected hosts, and are often excreted in feces. They range in size from tiny, single-celled organisms to worms that are visible to the naked eye. Their lifecycle may also vary. While some parasites use a permanent host, others go through a series of developmental phases using different animal or human hosts.

The illnesses they can cause range from mild discomfort to debilitating illness and even death. Parasites may be transmitted from host to host through consumption of contaminated food and water, or by putting anything into your mouth that has touched the stool (feces) of an infected person or animal.

Half of the world's population may have a protozoan parasite, Toxoplasma gondii, which scientists now believe may have a terrible influence on human behavior. Laboratory tests and a new report suggest that this parasite may cause or intensify severe forms of schizophrenia, impact how human hormones are secreted in the brain, and even cause personality changes. Scientists have determined that this parasite, which thrives in rats and reproduces in house cats, tricks rats into getting into harm's way. "The parasite grows in a rodent, but it needs to get into a cat somehow to reproduce," says Shelley Adamo, a biologist who studies neuroparasitology at Dalhousie University in Halifax, Canada. "When a rat becomes infected, the parasite somehow makes rats become attracted to cat urine, which it would normally avoid." Thus, the parasite tricks its host into suicide in order to reproduce.

The CDC estimates that more than sixty million Americans carry this same parasite. Most people get it from infected, undercooked meat, or from contact with cats. According to the agency, "Of those who are infected, very few have symptoms because a healthy person's immune system usually keeps the parasite from causing illness." But scientists are starting to rethink that theory.

In 1896, *Scientific American* ran an editorial entitled "Is insanity due to a microbe?" and thus started a lively discussion on infectious causes of schizophrenia, epilepsy, and other diseases of the mind. But why does 'science' take over a hundred years to try to answer a simple question? I remember a gritty crime movie called *Serpico*. In *Serpico*, Al Pacino plays the part of an honest cop who is trying to cope with the rampant and widespread corruption of his colleagues in the New York Police force. It's a confronting and tense drama—one that saw Pacino nominated for an Academy Award for Best Actor in 1974.

In this movie, there is a dramatic scene in which Serpico and his girlfriend, Laurie, are talking about his dilemma. The following story is told:

"Did you ever hear the story of the Wise King?"
"Nope, but I got the feeling I'm gonna hear it."
"Well, there was this king, and he ruled over his kingdom. Right in the middle of the kingdom there was a well. That's where everybody drank.

One night, this witch came along . . . and she poisoned the well (with pollution and Toxoplasma gondii) . . . And the next day, everybody drank from it except the king . . . and they all went crazy. They got together in the street and they said . . . 'We got to get rid of the king, 'cause the king is mad.'

And then that night, the king went down and he drank from the well. And the next day all the people rejoiced . . . because their king had regained his reason."

We live in a very polluted world and we are constantly accumulating toxins from our air, water, and food until we have all become intoxicated. If you then add parasites and pressure to the equation, you may begin to understand why the entire world seems to have gone "nuts!" Billions of intoxicated people all over the world need to detox and cleanse themselves of toxins and parasites!

There are many ways to remove parasites that we will cover in this book, and it is up to you to decide which cleanse is right for you. Some cleanses are more difficult to carry out than others. However, the goal of each parasite cleansing protocol remains the same: to kill and eliminate the parasites from your body.

Let us now look at the various ways to safely and effectively eliminate your parasites.

CHAPTER 1

The Best Parasite Cleansing Methods

The most common parasite infestation problems lie within your own digestive system. Parasites in food require an incubation period of 36 hours. You should have a bowel movement to eliminate the waste from whatever you eat within 16 to 24 hours. But, the average elimination time in America today is *96 hours.*

If waste is not eliminated within 24 hours, it begins a toxic buildup and creates a perfect breeding ground for parasitic infections. A clogged intestine with putrid fecal matter and plenty of sugar (which Americans consume far too much of today) provides the ideal environment for parasites to thrive. It is now common knowledge that the average American adult has between 10 to 20 pounds of waste rotting in their intestines. In the words of *National Geographic,* this waste material is home to "a sinister world of monstrous creatures that feed on living flesh—parasites."

Discover published a feature article in its August 2000 issue stating:

"Every living thing has at least one parasite that lives inside or on it, and many, including humans, have far more. Scientists are only just beginning to discover exactly how powerful these hidden inhabitants can be, but their research is pointing to a remarkable possibility: parasites may rule the world. The notion that tiny creatures we've largely taken for granted are such a dominant force is immensely disturbing. We are collections of cells that work together, kept harmonized by chemical signals. If an organism can control those signals—an organism like a parasite—then it can control us—and therein lies the peculiar and precise horror of parasites."

Not even cooking can kill all of the parasite eggs! People who say they don't believe they could possibly have parasites are naïve; parasites are everywhere.

We "worm" our pets and animals regularly. Shouldn't we at least take the same precautions to deworm ourselves and our families?

Diatomaceous Earth

I suggest you, your family, and pets all eat one tablespoon of food-grade diatomaceous earth (DE) mixed in water for at least seven consecutive days, at least twice per year, to help remove parasites and worms.

Diatomaceous earth is the best natural anti-parasitic medication that I have ever researched, studied, or used. Food-grade DE does not harm humans or pets. DE is believed to kill insects, worms, and parasites by dehydrating them. One tablespoon taken by an adult once a day for seven days is extremely effective at killing most parasites.

If this is going to be given to children, bear in mind that height is a better indicator of the size of their gastrointestinal tract than their weight. Thus, a child who is four feet tall should take two teaspoons, and a child who is two feet tall should take one teaspoon. Make sure only to use plain food-grade DE. Some DE has synthetic pesticides added to it. Industrial diatomaceous earth is used for swimming pool filters—this type of DE has been chemically treated, and neither type of non-food grade DE is safe for you to eat.

Try to avoid rubbing a lot of DE onto your hands, as it can have a drying effect on your skin. Do not breathe any form of DE or any fine dust, as it can irritate your lungs. Diatomaceous earth contains heavy metals as part of its mineral content, but it also contains the natural antidote selenium, which allows otherwise accumulative heavy metals to be flushed from the body. Therefore, it is not really a health concern despite the presence of minute amounts of naturally occurring aluminum and lead. I recommend taking one 400 mcg selenium supplement a day for at least a week after discontinuing any food-grade DE cleanse or treatment to ensure that your body thoroughly flushes out all of the heavy metals. My research indicates that diatomaceous earth is the best overall parasite treatment for humans because it should also kill all microscopic blood-borne parasites as well. When using DE, be sure to drink plenty of fluids, because it may dehydrate you.

Bentonite Clay

Bentonite (montmorillonite) and other clays (aided by psyllium and flaxseed) will help your gut to detoxify by adsorbing disease-causing bacteria, viruses, mold, parasites, etc. and carrying them out of your body in your feces. When you choose to use bentonite clays as an "intestinal broom," remember that they don't just carry out the bad bacteria, but also all the good bacteria.

Clay cannot distinguish between species of microorganism. It just adsorbs it all and carries it out! The value of montmorillonite (the active ingredient in Bentonite) lies in its ability to adsorb (not absorb) many times its own weight and volume in a liquid medium. It has a predominantly negative charge that is capable of attracting many kinds of positively charged particles. Bentonite clay's structure helps it attract and soak up toxins and contaminants on its exterior wall, then draw them into the interior center of the clay, where they are held and then excreted out in your stool. It is this sponge-like quality of the Bentonite Clay that makes it a good anti-diarrhea substance, as it detoxes your body!

If your bacterial flora is unhealthy, soaking up the bad flora is a good thing. But, if you're supplementing with probiotics and trying to implant a healthy bacterial flora, then you may not want to ingest large amounts of a substance that's going to pull all those good bacteria out of your gut as well.

If you use bentonite clay on its own (in substantial amounts), it absorbs a lot of water and so can be used to stop diarrhea, or in people with normal bowel function, it can cause constipation. But, when used in smaller amounts and in combination with stool bulking/softening agents like freshly ground flaxseed and/or psyllium, it can actually relieve constipation because it makes your stools soft and spongy, stimulating peristalsis and making them easier to pass. Either way, bentonite clay helps you avoid hemorrhoids, which is a huge benefit.

Bentonite clay is a clay that is derived from volcanic ash deposits. Although bentonite is found in a variety of clays, calcium bentonite—also known as montmorillonite or pascalite—is historically considered to be the safest and most beneficial clay for use as a treatment for various health problems. Ancient cultures across the globe—from the Africans to native South American tribes, to the Aborigines and the Greeks and Romans—used bentonite clay to treat conditions such as rashes, poisoning, diarrhea, dysentery, and infections of the skin and mouth. I use hydrated bentonite clay to externally relieve the pain of stings and bites, and have often hydrated the clay with colloidal silver.

Animals also use clay for health reasons. All sorts of macaws converge at a small area on the main clay lick outside the Tambopata Research Center in the Peruvian Amazon rainforest. The clay lick is pretty much a simple cliff face. Somehow all of the birds know that the clay they eat in the morning will dispel the toxins in the poisonous fruit during the day. They only need to eat clay during the times of the year when the non-poisonous fruit is not available. Many species of parrot know to do this. How do they all know? When did they learn? How did they discover this amazing ability of the clay to remove poisons, and propagate it to the rest of the parrots? No one knows for sure, but we know it works!

When it is ingested, bentonite clay is thought to display a number of properties that make it an effective method for collecting and ridding the body of accumulated parasites as it passes through the intestinal tract. One of these properties is that, as the clay absorbs water in the digestive system, each of the clay's particles swells, forming a large, porous mass. As this indigestible mass moves through the intestinal tract, it is believed that the strong negative charge on its outer molecules attracts and drags along with it toxins, pathogenic viruses, and all types of parasites attached to the intestinal tissue's walls. When you use bentonite clay as an intestinal parasite cleanser, it's recommended that you also use it with freshly ground flaxseed or psyllium husk powder. The bentonite clay is thought to absorb the toxins and parasites, while the psyllium husk or flaxseed powder prevents constipation by providing a large amount of indigestible fiber to keep the mass moving through the intestinal tract and out of the body.

To begin a month-long bentonite parasite cleanse, combine one teaspoon of clay and one teaspoon of psyllium husk powder (or freshly ground flaxseed) in water and stir to blend. Drink the entire glass, then drink another glass of plain water. Continue to follow this pattern, drinking the clay-psyllium (clay-flaxseed) mixture either two hours before or two hours after eating, for three days. Drink the mixture twice on days four and five, and three times on the sixth day. After this point, finish out the month by consuming the mixture four times a day.

Calcium bentonite clay is a natural de-wormer. It gently removes parasites from the intestinal tract and safely eliminates them, all without the use of harmful chemicals or medications. In addition, the clay also cleanses the digestive tract of bad bacteria, viruses, and fungi, which allows you or your animals to better absorb nutrients. This detoxifying action also aids you or your pet's liver and kidneys, which can easily become overloaded with toxins. Hydrated bentonite clay works wonders for many different skin ailments including scabies, mange, cuts, abrasions, rashes, and hot spots.

Made into a poultice and applied directly to the skin, the clay acts as an analgesic (meaning it quickly reduces pain and itching). It speeds the healing process by pulling out bacteria that can cause infections or rashes. It can even reduce the chance of scar tissue development. In addition, the clay is non-toxic and perfectly safe! You can hydrate bentonite clay for external use with colloidal silver. Colloidal silver kills germs of all kinds, including bacteria, viruses, microbes, yeast, molds, spores, and other pathogens that can cause serious illness and disease. Colloidal silver is so safe and non-toxic that it can be used in a newborn baby's eyes moments after birth as an anti-bacterial to kill pathogens introduced during birth. In Ghana, colloidal silver is used to treat malaria, tuberculosis, gonorrhea, fungal skin infections, vaginal infections, urinary tract infections, tonsillitis, pharyngitis, conjunctivitis (pink eye), upper respiratory tract infections, and nasal and sinus problems.

Bentonite clay is non-toxic and cannot be absorbed by the intestinal tract. Proponents of its use claim that you can not only cure a large number of digestive system dysfunctions with regular cleanses, but that the amount of vitamins and minerals you can absorb will increase following a bentonite clay cleanse. However, because the clay includes small amounts of aluminum, anyone with an aluminum allergy or sensitivity should avoid using a bentonite cleanse. Bentonite cleanses should also not be used too often, since the clay can cause beneficial nutrients to be eliminated from the body. Bentonite clay is usually sold as a thick, tasteless, light-gray gel, but can also come in a powder or capsule form. It is best to take the clay when your stomach is empty. It can also be taken at least one hour before or after a meal, or right before going to sleep at night. Remember to add some freshly ground flaxseed or psyllium.

In *Cleansing the Body and the Colon for a Happier and Healthier You* by Teresa Schumacher and Toni Schumacher Lund, the authors state that a clogged-up colon and its parasitic infection is often the undiagnosed root of many physical problems. But, Schumacher writes, the medical profession *"does not even agree with the notion of filthy and impacted colons contributing to American ill health. This may be because there are no patented drugs for quick relief of impacted colons. The only way to cleanse intestines is with natural ingredients, and via a persistent personal hygiene program."*

In his book, *The Clay Cure*, Ran Knishinsky writes:

"While many herbs and homeopathic remedies are suggested for this condition, I believe clay offers one of the finest treatments for all types of parasites. First, its use will stimulate the gall bladder to increase the flow of bile according to Raymond Dextreit, a French naturopath. He writes that no parasite can live too long under any bilious condition. Second, considerable research has shed light on the connection between clay eating and parasites. The American Journal of Clinical Nutrition mentions this in a recent article: 'Geophagy (the practice of eating earthy or soil-like substances such as clay, and chalk) can be a source of nutrients. Its primary way of enhancing nutritional status appears to be, however, to counter dietary toxins and, secondarily, the effects of gastrointestinal parasites' (Johns and Duquette 1991).

Further, numerous citations in a host of other journals collaborate this fact: throughout the globe, people eat clay in response to parasites. Third, worms are themselves clay-eaters and are attracted to clay. As a result, when the clay is eliminated from the body, so are the worms. But the process isn't quick; for every worm eliminated several worm eggs are usually left behind. However, as the eggs hatch, the new worms are also immediately attracted to the clay, and in time, the entire problem should be disposed of."

Knishinsky recommends ingesting clay daily. To do this, you can either eat hydrated clay or drink liquefied clay. Generally, it is suggested that one to two tablespoons of hydrated clay is the proper daily amount for an adult. For those who prefer to take their clay in liquid form, we recommend one to two ounces daily. In all three cases, it is recommended to take the clay on an empty stomach for best results. And if you're taking any medication, it is recommended you wait one to three hours before ingesting clay, but please check with your physician, as medications vary in time release and content.

Note: When you complete any cleanse, you need to take a probiotic to replace the good bacteria in your gut.

CHAPTER 2

Fasting Cleanses

A green vegetable juice fast is a great way to rid the body of parasites. Not only do green juices help to eliminate the infestation and toxins, but they are also rich in vitamins and other nutrients that help to strengthen your immune system. A strong immune system is better able to protect your body against any type of infestation. Cucumbers, tomatoes, broccoli, celery, green peppers, leafy greens, lemons, ginger, and other herbs and spices are excellent foods for making green juices. Garlic and onions are also effective against parasites and can be juiced along with the vegetables.

Since the juice is stripped of all its fiber, there is no digestion going on, which means the bowels are prone to stop several days into the fast. It is important that the bowels are encouraged to continue moving in order to expel the dead parasites and other toxins that are present. This can be done by taking psyllium, triphala, freshly ground flax seed, magnesium, or any mild laxative on a daily basis. Senna is also a laxative that can be taken, but it is rather harsh and should not be used for more than three days as the body can become dependent on it. A juice fast is able to offer your body plenty of nutrients and can therefore be carried out for as long as needed or as long as your body is able to stick with it.

A lemon juice cleanse is another effective way to expel the parasites from the body. Lemon juice has a natural cleansing effect on your body that not only cleanses your intestinal tract, but can also cleanse your body at a deeper cellular level. As a result, the unwanted parasites are eventually starved because they cannot feed in a clean environment. Another benefit of lemon juice is that it is high in vitamin C. Vitamin C is a powerful antioxidant that helps to strengthen and build up your immune system.

Fasting is one of the oldest and most common methods of detoxification known to man. According to Joel Fuhrman, MD, in his book, *Fasting and Eating For Health*: "*The fast does not merely detoxify; it also breaks down superfluous tissue, fat, abnormal cells, atheromatous plaque and tumors, and releases diseased tissues and their cellular products into the circulation for elimination. Toxic or unwanted materials circulate in our bloodstream and lymphatic tissues, and are deposited in and released from our fat stores and other tissues. An important element of fasting detoxification is mobilizing the toxins from their storage areas."*

Drinking plenty of water and juice is effective in more ways than one when attempting a cleanse. The most obvious benefit is their helpfulness in carrying away unwanted toxins that were mobilized during the fasting process and removing them from your body. They are also important in preventing dehydration during this process. Also, many juices contain sugars that can assist in speeding up elimination. Juices can also be a good natural source of vitamins and minerals that your body needs to stay healthy and keep its energy during the cleansing process.

The symptoms of detoxification may include headaches and other aches and pains, fatigue, mood swings, weight loss, sleep disorders, and digestive problems. Any mild or moderate symptoms such as these should be welcomed because they are a sign that your body is healing and eliminating stored toxins. After any proper cleanse, you should maintain a diet that is both anti-parasite and anti-infection. Foods like garlic, pumpkin seeds, pomegranate juice, apple cider vinegar, cayenne pepper, cinnamon, cloves and probiotic yogurt can be incorporated into your daily diet so that you can make your intestines inhospitable to many parasites.

Because processed and cooked foods tend to create or add to the toxins in your colon, a cleanse consisting of mostly organic raw fruits and vegetables is your best bet for cleaning out your system. Organic raw fruits and vegetables are high in fiber, which is possibly the safest way to remove unwanted toxins from your digestive tract. Also, they contain the vitamins, minerals, amino acids, and enzymes necessary for a healthy body, so you won't feel weak or unwell as you're cleansing yourself. Avoiding all refined foods, sugars, and dairy products is a good idea to avoid feeding parasites. Eat high-fiber foods to not only get rid of worms, but to create an environment that is inhospitable to all parasites. When you are going through a parasite cleanse program, increase your water intake to more effectively eliminate the parasites from your body. Be sure to maintain frequent bowel movements during this time. Support bowel function with fiber, acidophilus, aloe vera, magnesium, and if needed, natural laxatives.

CHAPTER 3

Types of Intestinal Parasites

The two main types of intestinal parasites are helminths and protozoa. Helminths are worms with many cells. Tapeworms, pinworms, and roundworms are among the most common helminths in the United States. In their adult form, helminths cannot multiply in the human body. Protozoa have only one cell, and can multiply inside the human body, which can allow serious infections to develop. Intestinal parasites are usually transmitted when someone comes in contact with infected feces (for example, through contaminated soil, food, or water). In the U.S., the most common protozoa are giardia (beaver fever) and cryptosporidium.

Tapeworms

Obtaining a beef or pork parasite is rather easy, but also easily avoidable. Undercooked meat is a common way to ingest both Taenia solium and Taenia saginata tapeworms, whose larvae often live inside pigs and cows. Either species of tapeworm can grow up to twelve feet and live inside of a human host for several years. Tapeworms can cause a variety of health problems, including seizures, obscured or blurry vision, and a swelling of the brain if larvae move to that region. Most infections are asymptomatic, however, with the patient only realizing they are harboring a tapeworm when they pass a wiggling section of the worm while defecating. Manual removal of a tapeworm through the mouth is also possible, but not fun. It sounds incredible, but in the early 1900s a "nutrient absorption" product appeared. "No diet, no baths, no exercise. FAT—the enemy that is shortening your life—BANISHED." How? With sanitized tapeworms—jar-packed! How insane to use tapeworms to lose weight!

Hookworms

Hookworms lay traps in the soil. The hookworm is much smaller than a tapeworm. These parasites are rarely more than a centimeter long and burrow into your small intestine to feast on your blood. Since hookworms latch onto your small intestine and divert nutrients away from the bloodstream, they're actually more problematic than tapeworms. Hookworm infection can lead to anemia, slower cognitive growth, and malnutrition. Hookworms infect over a billion people worldwide.

The vast majority of these people live without advanced sanitation, amidst subtropical and tropical climates. Transmission of hookworms is quite devious and more involved than tapeworm transmission. When the soil cools off at night, hookworm larvae extend out of the soil, waiting to latch onto any human foot that passes overhead. Local sanitation problems come into the equation when larvae are passed through feces, allowing them to infect humans through both direct contact and contaminated water.

Pinworms

Pinworms sneak out of your anus at night! Tiny pinworms lay eggs around a host's anus, leading to an itching sensation, which creates a vicious cycle if your fingers come in contact with your mouth, since this allows the eggs to enter your digestive tract. Pinworms are found worldwide, and they're the bane of many North American elementary schools, as infections often begin through human contact or through recently used surfaces like toilet seats, faucets, and doorknobs.

Thankfully, the symptoms of a pinworm infection are not nearly as severe as a hookworm invasion. The worst pinworm symptoms include itchiness, irritability, and weight loss. A common test for pinworms involves taping the anal region of a possible host and inspecting the tape for eggs after a good night's sleep (if you can sleep in that condition). Pinworms don't just travel to the anus and lay eggs as part of a cruel joke—they need access to fresh air for their eggs to mature.

Giardia

Giardia infection can occur through ingestion of dormant microbial cysts in contaminated water, food, or by the fecal-oral route (through poor hygiene practices). The cyst can survive for weeks to months in cold water, so it can be present in contaminated wells and water systems, especially stagnant water sources, such as naturally occurring ponds, storm water storage systems, and even clean-looking mountain streams. They may also occur in city reservoirs and persist after water treatment, as the cysts are resistant to conventional water treatment methods, such as chlorination and ozonolysis. Zoonotic transmission is also possible, so Giardia infection is a concern for people camping in the wilderness or swimming in contaminated streams or lakes, especially the artificial lakes formed by beaver dams (hence the popular name for giardiasis, "beaver fever").

In addition to waterborne sources, fecal-oral transmission can also occur, for example in day-care centers, where children may have poor hygiene practices. Those who work with children are also at risk of being infected, as are family members of infected individuals. Not all Giardia infections are symptomatic, and many people can unknowingly serve as carriers of the parasite.

Cryptosporidium

Cryptosporidium infection is a gastrointestinal disease whose primary symptom is diarrhea. The illness begins when the tiny cryptosporidium parasites enter your body and travel to your small intestine. Cryptosporidium then begins its life cycle inside your body, burrowing into the walls of your intestines and then later being shed in your feces. In most healthy people, a cryptosporidium infection produces a bout of watery diarrhea, and the infection usually goes away within a week or two.

If you have a compromised immune system, a cryptosporidium infection can become life-threatening without proper treatment. You can help prevent cryptosporidium by practicing good hygiene and by avoiding water that hasn't been boiled or filtered.

CHAPTER 4

Signs and Symptoms of Parasite Infestations

Stomach & Intestinal Complications

Symptoms of an infestation may include:

- ➢ Persistent diarrhea
- ➢ Chronic constipation
- ➢ Gas & Bloating
- ➢ Digestive problems
- ➢ Excessive early bowel movements (very explosive bowel movements very soon after eating)
- ➢ Abdominal pain
- ➢ Mucus in the stool
- ➢ Leaky gut
- ➢ Chronic, unexplained nausea, often accompanied by vomiting
- ➢ Intestinal cramping
- ➢ Hemorrhoids
- ➢ Dysentery (loose stools containing blood and mucus)
- ➢ Urinary Tract Infections
- ➢ Rash or itching around the rectum or vulva
- ➢ Burning in the stomach

- Foul-smelling gas
- Indigestion
- Bloating
- Bloody stool and in severe cases coughing blood
- Fatigue
- Chronic Fatigue Syndrome
- Low energy
- Lethargy and excessive weakness

Skin Disorders & Allergies

Symptoms include:

- Dry skin
- Dry or brittle hair
- Hair loss
- AllergiesItchy ears, nose, eyes, skin, soles of the feet, or anus
- Hives
- Allergic reactions to food
- Chronic ear and/or sinus infections
- Crawling sensation under the skin
- Rashes
- Weeping Eczema
- Cutaneous ulcers
- Papular lesions
- Swelling
- Sores
- Facial swelling around the eyes (roundworms) and wheezing

and coughing, followed by vomiting, stomach pain, and bloating (suggesting roundworms or threadworms)

Mood & Anxiety Problems

➢ Mood swings

➢ Unexplained dizziness

➢ Nervousness

➢ Depression

➢ Forgetfulness

➢ Unclear thinking

➢ Restlessness

➢ Anxiety

➢ Slow reflexes

Sleep Disturbances

➢ Insomnia

➢ Teeth grinding during sleep

➢ Difficulty sleeping

➢ Bed wetting

➢ Drooling while asleep

➢ Disturbed sleep with multiple awakenings

Weight & Appetite Problems

Parasites rob the body of all essential nutrients (they get the choicest nutrition from the food you eat) and you are left with the fats, sugars, etc. Many overweight people are infested with parasites. They stay hungry, which leads to overeating because of the parasites. Depending on the type of parasite infestation, many people become malnourished and they can't gain weight, again, because of the parasites. This is why parasites cause weight gain, long-standing obesity, loss of appetite or uncontrollable hunger, eating more than normal but still feeling hungry, and the inability to gain or lose weight.

Muscle & Joint Complaints

Muscle pain; joint pain; muscle cramping; numbness of the hands and/or feet; heart pain; pain in the navel; pain in the back, thighs, or shoulders; arthritic pains; palpitations (hookworms); and fast heartbeat.

Blood Disorders

Hypoglycemia and Anemia.

Sexual & Reproductive Problems

- ➢ Male impotence
- ➢ Erectile dysfunction
- ➢ PMS
- ➢ Candida (yeast infections)
- ➢ Urinary tract infections
- ➢ Cysts & fibroids
- ➢ Menstrual problems
- ➢ Prostate problems
- ➢ Water retention

These things will raise your risk for getting intestinal parasites:

- ➢ Lack of personal protection and proper concern
- ➢ Ignorance of proper hygiene

- ➤ Living in or visiting an area known to have parasites
- ➤ International travel, especially to third world countries
- ➤ Poor sanitation (for both food and water)
- ➤ Poor hygiene—wash your hands and clean under your fingernails
- ➤ Age—children and the elderly are more likely to get infected
- ➤ Exposure to child and institutional care centers
- ➤ Improper diet
- ➤ Having a weakened immune system (e.g., HIV or AIDS) or immune-suppressing drugs

There are a number of simple ways to avoid getting infected with parasites, such as preparing your own food, properly washing fruits and vegetables, washing your hands before eating and after using the bathroom, wearing socks or shoes instead of going barefoot, and keeping your fingernails short and clean.

CHAPTER 5

How Do I Get Rid Of My "Bugs"?

You should see your doctor and ask for a complete parasitic panel, including stool study if you have symptoms of chronic inflammation or poor digestion. There are antibiotics that treat parasites. However, most parasites will quickly grow back from the remaining eggs if you do not follow the proper procedures.

There are natural remedies that give relief from parasites, killing them and their eggs. There are also holistic treatments that can knock out the parasitic infection with strong herbs. See your local herbalist for evaluation, especially if antibiotics are not right for you.

Ginger is a good staple to keep in your diet for removing and preventing parasitic infestations. It has long been used in Africa and India to treat parasites. Look also for antiparasitic herbs, such as wormwood bark, to treat common parasite infestations. It is also important to have regular bowel movements. A bowel movement should occur every time you eat. A minimum of two bowel movements a day is healthy. Less than one movement a day means you are constipated. Eat plenty of fiber and cleanse at least twice a year to keep your digestive health moving. Ayurvedic triphala (literally "three fruits") powder is one of the few beneficial laxatives I recommend for occasional use. Laxatives should never be used for more than seven days in a row.

If a conventional doctor believes that you have parasites, he/she will prescribe you an anti-parasitic pharmaceutical. These pharmaceuticals are always toxic, for it is their toxicity that kills the parasites. Thus, swelling of your lymph nodes, hands, and feet is common, and vision problems, lack of coordination, and convulsions can also occur. Diarrhea is a typical side effect with these drugs. I experience no parasite infestations as long as I periodically eat food-grade DE.

Herbs for Getting Rid of Intestinal Parasites

The following foods, herbs, supplements, and dietary recommendations may also be part of your treatment or cleanse program to remove and control intestinal parasites.

1) Garlic (Allium sativa) has been found to have activity against Ascaris (roundworm), Giardia lamblia, Trypanosoma, Plasmodium, and Leishmania. Garlic is available in capsule and tablet form, as well as whole garlic cloves. Garlic contains allicin, which has been shown to get rid of parasites in both test tubes and animal studies. Eating garlic has been known to kill parasites. When using garlic to treat parasites, it is best to eat it before meals. Doing so will stimulate gastric secretions and kill off the invaders.

2) Goldenseal (Hydrastis Canadensis) has been used historically for infections involving the mucous membranes in the body, such as respiratory tract infections. Preliminary lab studies suggest that berberine, the active constituent of goldenseal, is active against Entamoeba histolytica, Giardia lamblia, and Plasmodium.

3) Black walnut is a folk herbal remedy used for ringworm and athlete's foot. The juice of unripe hulls of black walnut are used for parasites and fungal infections. The juice that is found in the green hulls of this herb is effective against parasites such as ringworm, and fungal infections like athlete's foot. According to expert Dr. Hulda Clark, if the hull has ripened and turned black, it is useless as an agent against parasites. In many cases, parasite-fighting tinctures are made with black walnut, wormwood, and clove oil.

4) Wormwood (Artemesia annua) has been used for centuries as an herbal remedy for intestinal parasites, especially against Ascaris lumbricoides, Plasmodium, Schistosoma mansoni, and Giardia. Wormwood contains sesquiterpene lactones, which are thought to weaken parasite membranes. Wormwood can be found in tea, liquid extract, or capsule form. However, the pure oil is considered toxic and should not be ingested. The safety and effectiveness of this herb has not been established in clinical trials.

5) Wormseed (Chenopodium ambrosioides) is a traditional herbal remedy used in the tropics for expelling roundworms, hookworms, and tapeworms. Concentrated wormseed oil is too potent to use, so many herbalists consider wormseed tea to be preferable. More scientific studies are needed to confirm the historical usage of this herb and its safety.

6) Pumpkin seeds (Curcubita pepo) or Mexican pepitas (pumpkin seeds rich in zinc) have been used as a remedy for tapeworms and roundworms. Herbalists often recommend large amounts (up to 25 ounces for adults). The seeds are often mashed and mixed with juice or yogurt. Two or three hours after consuming the pumpkin seeds, a laxative is often recommended to help cleanse the intestines.

Pumpkin seeds are known for their nutritional content and their ability to get rid of intestinal parasites. Roasted pumpkin seeds are not only a great snack, but the University of Maryland Medical Center also recommends consuming them (along with plenty of fluids) to help protect against and eliminate any parasites you may have. Pumpkin seeds are easy to eat with or without the shells, and it's easy to incorporate them in your meals or consume them as a snack. You can use them as a delicious topping for salads, a garnish for casseroles, or in breakfast cereals. Eating raw organic pumpkin seeds has been an effective way to kill and eliminate many kinds of parasites for years in Native American cultures. They are relatively inexpensive, and since they are one of the better tasting herbal remedies, they are a good choice for children. Tapeworms are just one of many parasites that have been removed by eating pumpkin seeds. Pepitas are also a very good source of magnesium, which is essential for easy bowel movements.

Importantly, this pumpkin seed remedy for intestinal worms does not actually kill the worms outright. It is believed the high levels of cucurbitins, and perhaps other unidentified compounds, actually paralyze the worms. This prevents them from holding on to the intestinal walls, as they usually do during a bowel movement. It is strongly recommended you follow this pumpkin seed worm treatment with a quick-acting laxative like castor oil to make sure that as many worms as possible are expelled into the toilet before they can recover.

7) Thyme is especially beneficial in the treatment of parasites found in the intestinal tract, such as tapeworms. Thyme contains a compound known as thymol, which prevents the growth of many parasites, including ringworm. Hookworms and roundworms have also been destroyed with the use of this herb.

8) Grapefruit seed has been shown in studies by the U.S. Food and Drug Administration to be effective at killing parasites and creating an environment in the body that stops their growth. Parasites cannot build up a resistance to a natural food like grapefruit seed extract. Because it is not toxic to the human body, it makes an excellent remedy for children and adults alike. It has no side effects and works against worms, protozoa, and fungal infections.

9) Diet change: Temporarily avoid coffee, refined sugar, alcohol, and refined foods, as they help feed many common parasites.

10) Intestinal cleansing involves the use of a higher-fiber diet plus supplements such as psyllium husks, citrus pectin, papaya extract, bentonite clay, activated charcoal, pumpkin seeds, beet root, and/or flaxseeds.

11) Other natural remedies: Anise, cloves, gentian, neem, olive leaf, oregano, propolis, thyme, barberry, Oregon grape, and cayenne pepper mixed in water will kill nematodes, so purify your drinking water with cayenne and/or place some cayenne pepper in a time release capsule to control nematodes in you. Pomegranates are useful for destroying worms in the intestinal tract. Eat them raw in isolation of your regular meals.

12) Citrus: If you have worms, try eating nothing but citrus fruits and other fruits high in citric acid for a week. The citric acid in the fruit kills worms and other parasites in the body. Such fruits (to be eaten fresh) are tomatoes, oranges, lemons, limes, grapefruits, and pineapples.

13) Onion and garlic juice: With every meal, juice half of a fresh onion and several cloves of garlic through a vegetable juicer. Mix the juice with half a cup of water and drink. This kills the parasites and worms in the system.

14) Apple cider vinegar: Three times daily, drink a cup of water mixed with three tablespoons of apple cider vinegar or plain white vinegar. The acid in the vinegar can kill the worms and parasite in the intestines.

15) Grind fresh ginger root to a pulp and mix with half a cup of water. Drink three times daily, and eat the pulp as well. It's very spicy but it will kill many types of parasites.

16) Papaya contains a substance called papain, which is a digestive enzyme. By consuming it 30 minutes before meals, it will help the environment inside your gut become unfriendly to parasites. Digestive enzymes help restore your intestinal tract to a balanced state, which makes it inhospitable to parasites.
Papaya seeds have been found to be effective against human intestinal parasites; the research was published in *The Journal of Medicinal Food*. In this study, a combination of papaya seeds and honey was fed to 30 children with intestinal parasites and after 7 days 23 of the 30 were cleared of the infestation.

17) Pineapples contain specific enzymes that target and destroy parasites. Both bromelain and papain are enzymes found in fresh pineapples that have protein-digesting attributes, which weakens the parasites and allows your body the chance to get rid of them.

18) Other herbs: The herbs best known for getting rid of parasites are thyme leaf, barberry, oregano, cloves, wormwood, and black walnut. Cloves kill the parasite eggs in the intestinal tract, and both black walnut hull and wormwood can eliminate about 100 types of these critters. Using fresh cloves is an effective remedy against parasitic infections. This may be why cloves historically are used when cooking ham. You can eat the fresh cloves as long as they have not been irradiated, as this destroys much of their effectiveness. The essential oil may also be used to dissolve the eggs left behind by worms found in the intestines. To date, this is the only herb that has been proven to destroy the eggs, which is one reason it is used in conjunction with other herbs such as black walnut to prevent a reinfestation.

19) Avoid sugar and starches: Parasites love sugar and everything that turns into sugar, so the best way to starve the parasites is through healthy fasting and cleansing strategies, while eliminating as much sugar and grains as possible (especially refined grains like white flour) from the diet.

20) Extra virgin coconut oil is loaded with medium chain triglycerides that support the immune system in its battle against parasites.

21) Dried oregano, and especially essential oil of oregano, are extremely volatile and anti-parasitic. Use two to three drops of oregano oil in water with freshly squeezed lemon and drink this three times a day. Clove oil works just as well, so you could also substitute or use clove oil with oregano oil. Please note that both oregano oil and clove oil are very strong and should never be eaten or come into contact with your skin without being diluted first.

22) Fasting with fermented drinks—such as fermented whey from grass-fed cows, fermented ginger, kombucha, coconut kefir, apple cider vinegar, etc.—are powerful tools to help destroy parasites. Many holistic health coaches recommend a 3 to 21-day low-calorie, liquid diet that is rich in fermented beverages, water, and freshly squeezed lemon.

23) Probiotic foods: After the cleansing period, it is especially important to utilize high-quality, fermented, raw dairy and vegetables. Raw, grass-fed fermented dairy products like amasai, cheese, and kimchi, as well as sauerkraut and fermented veggies should be used abundantly. These foods are rich sources of L-glutamine, an amino acid that helps rebuild the gut. These fermented foods also contain very powerful strains of good bacteria, organic acids, and enzymes that act to keep parasites out of the body.

24) Diatomaceous earth: I believe the very best way to control all parasites is by eating food-grade DE, especially on a "pulse therapy" basis. Pulse therapy means the administration of large doses of natural remedies in an intermittent manner to enhance the therapeutic effect and reduce any possible side effects.

Caution: A cat or dog is best treated with food-grade DE and/or pumpkin seed oil. Do not feed pets walnut hulls, wormwood, or any other supplement or food without first researching its side effects upon your pets. For instance, even a common food like an onion can kill a dog. Onions can cause a form of hemolytic anemia called Heinz body anemia in dogs, a condition that causes the destruction of red blood cells. Kidney damage may follow. Toxicity may occur from similar foods, such as garlic and chives. It is not clear what quantity of onions is poisonous, but the effects can be cumulative. Poisoning can result from raw, cooked, and dehydrated forms. Avoid feeding table scraps and any foods cooked with onions (including some baby foods).

Dogs also should not eat chocolate, grapes, raisins, avocados, macadamia nuts, caffeinated items, xylitol, alcohol, yeast dough, fruit pits, or seeds. Cats also should not eat onions in any form, nor should they be given aspirin, garlic, chives, dairy foods (as adults), any alcoholic drinks, grapes, raisins, caffeine, chocolate, xylitol, fat, raw eggs, meat, fish, yeast dough, and/or any human medicines.

25) Oil pulling is a safe, simple, cheap, and gentle 'do it yourself home remedy' that helps cure and prevent diseases and extends your healthy life. It involves gently rinsing the mouth with one tablespoon (10ml) of organic cold pressed oil for 15 to 20 minutes and spitting it out. You can use organic sunflower oil, sesame oil, or olive oil. This simple therapy is completely harmless, as you do not take any medicines (with side effects). Even the oil you use is never swallowed, but simply spit out after oil pulling. By helping the body get rid of toxins that have accumulated, oil pulling has been mentioned in the ancient texts of Ayurveda and promotes healing.

CHAPTER 6

The Elimination Phase

How will you feel as you cleanse your body of parasites? As parasites die, they release toxins through their excrement, and from rotting. Furthermore, many of the cleansing herbs and remedies in this book will also help remove toxins stored in your body and fat cells.

Be sure to maintain frequent bowel movements during this time to fully eliminate these toxins and prevent them from being reabsorbed in your body. Support bowel function with fiber, acidophilus, aloe vera, magnesium and natural laxatives if needed.

The most common worms may attempt to escape by burrowing deeper into your intestines, which can cause sharp pains and cramps. Even when dead, your body is still burdened with the task of flushing the dead parasites out. This whole process can initially make you feel sicker than before you started the cleanse! Realize this is only temporary, and it is a sign that the cleanse is really working.

While fatigue and grogginess are also to be expected, normal life may be continued, and diarrhea should not last more than a few days. Ensure that you are eating a good, wholesome diet throughout your cleanse to ensure that your immune system is at its strongest. After the cleanse, you should feel better, have more energy, and feel sick less often.

CHAPTER 7

Killing Parasitic Eggs and Worms in the Yard and Farms

Your yard may be a breeding ground for various parasites and worms, so it's important to learn what you can do to help remove these nasty invaders.

If you have dogs, clean any outdoor kennel area. Clean the kennel's floor surfaces with a solution of 1-2 ounces of Safe Solutions Tweetmint Enzyme Cleaner and 1/2 cup of borax per gallon of water. Steam clean the floors to kill any remaining eggs if you suspect there may be an infestation.

Remove all animal waste from the yard. Place animal waste in a garbage bag rather than tossing it on a compost pile, into shrubs, or any other location where parasites can reinfest the area. Prune back shade-giving structures such as trees or bushes in the yard. This will expose the yard to more direct sunlight. The direct sunlight is harmful to the worm eggs and will kill them over time. Finally, lightly spread diatomaceous earth in the yard. This substance may destroy the worm eggs and hatched worms may also eat it, which will kill them. In addition, the food-grade DE will also kill fleas.

Prevention is important! The common dog tapeworm can be controlled by eliminating fleas and lice from the environment. Dogs should be prevented from roaming and eating dead animals. Avoid feeding your dog uncooked meat and raw game. Echinococcus granulosa and Echinococcus multiocularis are both significant public health problems. Dogs and humans can acquire the infection from eating contaminated uncooked meat, and, in the case of dogs, by feeding on the carcass of an infected animal. Humans can also acquire the disease by ingesting eggs passed in the feces of dogs. Since humans are not the definitive host, adult worms do not develop. Instead, the larvae produce large cysts in your liver, lungs, and brain. These cysts are called hydatids, and they can cause serious illness and even death in people.

Echinococcus granulosus is found in the southern, western, and southwestern areas of the United States, where sheep and cattle are common. Although dog-to-human transmission is rare, a number of human cases (presumably from eating uncooked meat) are reported each year. If your dog runs free in a rural area where this tapeworm exists, ask your veterinarian to check your pet's stool for tapeworms twice a year.

This species of tapeworm can be identified only after the head has been recovered by effective deworming. Until a definite diagnosis is made, a dog with a tapeworm that could be Echinococcus must be handled with extreme care to avoid fecal contamination of your hands and food.

The cure to virtually all internal parasites is simple, safe, and effective. The governments of the United States and Canada both recognize that food-grade diatomaceous earth is safe to use in animal foods. Diatomaceous earth prevents "clumping" of feed particles by keeping them separate, so the surface area of feed exposed to the digestive processes, both bacterial and enzymatic, is increased and therefore more feed is actually digested and utilized. Diatomaceous earth contains a small amount of fifteen trace minerals. Thousands of animal owners and livestock breeders have discovered that adding diatomaceous earth to their animals' rations has produced a number of incredible benefits.

Diatomaceous earth is a remarkable, all-natural product made from tiny fossilized water plants. Diatomaceous earth is a naturally occurring siliceous sedimentary mineral compound from microscopic skeletal remains of unicellular, algae-like plants called diatoms. These plants have been part of the earth's ecology since prehistoric times. It is believed that thirty million years ago, the diatoms built up into deep, chalky deposits of diatomite. The diatoms are mined and ground up to render a powder that looks and feels like talcum powder to us. It is a mineral-based natural pesticide. DE is approximately 3% magnesium, 33% silicon, 19% calcium, 5% sodium, 2% iron, and contains many other trace minerals such as titanium, boron, manganese, copper, and zirconium.

Food-grade diatomaceous earth has been used for many years as a natural wormer for livestock. Some believe diatomaceous earth scratches and dehydrates parasites. Other scientists believe that diatomaceous earth is a de-ionizer or de-energizer of worms or parasites. Regardless of the theory, people report definite worm and parasite control.

To be most effective, food-grade diatomaceous earth must be fed long enough to catch all newly-hatching eggs or cycling of the worms through the lungs and back to the stomach. A minimum of 90 days is advised for lungworms. Food grade diatomaceous earth works in a purely physical and mechanical manner, not chemical, and thus has no chemical toxicity. Best yet, parasites will not build up a tolerance to its chemical reaction, so rotation of wormers is unnecessary. DE is also extremely effective on fleas, ticks, lice, and other insects, and can be applied to sleeping areas and rubbed into a pet's fur to prevent the fleas that carry tapeworm eggs.

A mixture of feed incorporating 2% diatomaceous earth was sent to three zoos for evaluation: John Ball Park of Grand Rapids, Michigan; Brookfield Zoo of Chicago, Illinois; and Buffalo Zoo of Buffalo, New York. John Ball and Buffalo Zoos reported that their black bears on the special feed showed a better coat and clearer eyes. The primates fed at the Brookfield Zoo displayed a pronounced improvement in both appearance and behavior. Stool samples taken at all three zoos showed an absence of any internal parasites (adults or eggs). Parasites in these animals were present prior to using the diatomaceous earth food mixture. A Bison rancher in Alberta conducted fecal test samples to check for parasites after using diatomaceous earth for several weeks. The tests came out negative. Neither he nor his vet believed it, so they took more samples from different Bison of different herds, which had been fed diatomaceous earth. The tests still came back negative.

Not only did he solve his parasite problem with a non-toxic, natural product, but he found that the coats and overall appearance of his bison had improved. Another benefit is that some diatomaceous earth remains in the manure, which prevents the eggs of flies and parasites from hatching out, thereby breaking the cycle of reinfestation. There were no maggots found in the manure with DE.

In her book *The Cure for All Cancers*, Dr. Hulda Clark implicates parasites as the root cause for most of the diseases inflicting the human species. As long as they remain in the intestines, our immune system can deal with them. When they are allowed to escape the intestines, they settle in the most vulnerable parts of our bodies. Dr. Clark states that cancer can be cured—not just treated—and after years of study, she discovered that many cancer patients have a certain parasite in their bodies. In clinical studies, she saw that after removing this parasite, the cancer stopped immediately, and the tissue returned to normal again.

Food-grade DE has been used for many years to deworm pets and has been used more recently in humans. With the ingestion of sushi and other raw types of seafood, or with eating undercooked meats or contaminated food products, there are more instances than ever of worms in humans. Most people do not realize the number of parasites that exist in their body, but this little book on parasites should help you understand that we are all loaded with them. Food-grade diatomaceous earth is safe for humans and their intestines.

I would like to note just one story of a cancer patient I have known. In 2005, a dear friend asked why I was eating food-grade DE, so I gave him one of my original articles on the subject. My friend read that I believed DE could help cure cancer, and asked if food-grade DE would harm another friend (with cancer) who had been given only four weeks to live by his oncologist. I said nothing could harm this cancer patient because he was simply "a dead man walking." I allowed my friend to take a bag of food-grade DE to "the dead man walking." About five months passed, and my friend reported that "the dead man walking" was still alive and his entire blood chemistry had been changed. Even so, the patient's oncologist demanded that his patient immediately stop taking food-grade DE. The oncologist then continued his cancer "treatments" until his patient died.

Parasites exist by robbing your body of nutrients. Parasites are the root cause of lupus, with all other symptoms being secondary to your parasitic infection. Lupus can be cured simply with a proper parasite cleanse. According to conventional doctors, lupus is thought to be an "incurable disease" and/or an "autoimmune disorder." Parasitic diseases are illnesses caused by infestation (infection) with parasites such as protozoa (one-celled animals), worms, or insects. Parasites often target vital organs and systems, altering the normal functions of the body. Thus, parasites play the role of a transmitter of some of medical science's most lethal diseases.

All Diatomaceous Earth (DE) is Not the Same.

Though it is all mined from the ground, diatomaceous earth (DE) is not an earth, but fossilized deposits of microscopic shells that are created by single one-celled plants called "diatoms." On land, the basic food for all land animals is grass. Those animals that do not eat grass eat the animals that do eat grass. The silica content of all living organisms is linked with the diet. Silica is highest for the pure plant eaters and lowest for the pure meat eaters. In all water, tiny one-celled plants or plankton live by the billions of billions of billions, and they are the basic food of the water-dwelling animals. Even the great whales could not survive without the tiny little diatoms. As these tiny creatures die, by the billions of billions of billions, their shells or exoskeletons drift to the bottom of the ocean or lake, building up large deposits. Each dead diatom exoskeleton now is a tiny piece of porous sand. Geologic changes eventually put these deposits on dry land, making them accessible to mankind.

Because of water currents, most DE deposits are very impure. Some even contain arsenic and can be very dangerous. Many people tend to think that all diatomaceous earth is the same, but nothing could be further from the truth. There is a great diversity of DE deposits, just as there is a great diversity of everything on the planet.

There are more than 25,000 species of diatoms, but only two primary types of diatomaceous earth deposits. Not all diatoms are aquatic; some exist in moist conditions, but since three-fourths of the earth is covered with oceans, most deposits are of the saltwater type. Just one liter of sea water may contain as many as ten million one-celled pieces of algae. There are deposits which also occur in freshwater lakes, and within this second type of deposit, the purity is exceptional.

While other insecticide poisons kill chemically as neurotoxins, the insect pests (over time) develop a resistance or an immunity to the chemicals. Food-grade DE kills bugs physically, and insects have not been known to develop immunity to its physical action. Food-grade DE is certain death to insects because it kills by actually puncturing the insect's exoskeleton, disrupting its soft waxy shell structure, chewing up its digestive organs, and causing death in a short time by dehydration. Add a little powdered sugar to attract pests to the DE.

How to Safely and Effectively Apply Food-Grade Diatomaceous Earth

There are many creatures that can bite you or your pets, including bed bugs, fleas, mites, spiders, ticks, etc. One of the easiest and most effective ways to control them all is with food-grade DE, First, you should thoroughly vacuum the infested areas (beds, furniture, and floors) to remove as many pests as possible. Then, put on a dust filter mask and turn the vacuum around so that the exhaust points towards these vacuumed areas. With food-grade DE in a pepper/salt shaker, lightly shake out some DE so that it will fall directly into the vacuum's exhaust stream for a few seconds. A very light cloud of DE will then be lightly applied all over the infested areas. Do not enter any area until the dust completely settles. You can clean up any unwanted residues from surfaces that are not suspected to be infested using a damp cloth. Properly applied DE either repels or kills most insects and arachnids and does not need not to be applied very often, so apply DE only as needed. IF YOU SEE WHITE IT IS NOT RIGHT, meaning you have used more DE than you need.

The DE particle scrapes, punctures, and tears into the body of the insect, causing a loss of fluid. Insects do not have blood vessels like higher forms of life. They have an exoskeleton (outer shell) that is semi-porous—more or less like unglazed porcelain. In order to keep their body fluids from evaporating through their shells, nature also puts a waxy coating on the outside. If you were to take a brand new shoeshine and put DE on one shoe, then leave it for 20 minutes before blowing it off, you would have no shine. The DE would have absorbed the wax. You have much the same situation with insects. Once the protective coating is gone, the insects slowly dehydrate. *National Geographic* tells about cockroaches that died within twelve hours after exposure to DE. DE also stops the breathing apparatus of insects. They ingest it and it lacerates them inside, and yet this same material, even if we accidentally inhale it, really doesn't damage a person all that much (no more than inhaling any fine dust would).

There were two vets who told me that there is only one worm, called Strongyles, that apparently diatomaceous earth does not kill, but it cleans out all the others. We have had treated beef cows go through slaughter. An affidavit was made to the effect that there were absolutely no internal parasites anywhere in those that had been fed food-grade DE. The microscopic shells in diatomaceous earth (DE) are composed of silicon dioxide and around fourteen trace minerals. Being formed under water, they will not dissolve in water. In fact, even in the stomach acid of animals or birds, surrounded with powerful digestive (acidic) juices, they pass all the way through the body, almost completely. A very small amount is leached out.

The shape of these shells and the size of the holes in their surface is very important. Many harmful things entering the body have a positive charge. Silica is a semi-conductive mineral which, when warmed by body heat, becomes negatively charged and gives off electrons. These negatively charged mineral ions and/or individual shells attract bad microbes, free radicals, positively charged waste, and other harmful things. Acting as magnets, the negatively charged shells and/or ions attract and absorb positive things that are small enough to go through the holes. Add a sugar molecule and you can trap toxins into the porous food-grade DE particle, which is then excreted safely out of your body. Because of the strong charge, each shell can absorb a large number of positively charged substances, whether they are chemical or in the form of bacteria or viruses. They pass on through your stomach and intestine, taking all these harmful substances out of your body.

In today's world, most all food (animal or human), water, and air contain harmful substances, which when taken internally, cause stress on the immune system, wasting energy that could go toward the production of milk or meat. For example, Dr. Johnson, a Canadian veterinarian, discovered that DE absorbs the bacteria, causing "scours" (diarrhea). The DE takes them out of the body and the animal is protected from unnecessary stress and possible death. Passing through the digestive system, food-grade DE rubs against parasites and, being very abrasive, causes serious damage, leading the parasite to die and pass out of the animals with no negative side effects. The effect on the animal is nothing but beneficial. Most living creatures are in contact with parasite eggs and toxic substances on a daily basis.

Having food-grade DE in the diet every day tends to keep the animal free of parasites and toxic chemicals so it can get maximum benefits from the food and water it consumes. Vet bills tend to be reduced by around 75%. I've also been told a heaping teaspoon of food-grade DE in yogurt or orange juice will cure E. coli.

Here's how to feed food-grade Diatomaceous Earth to your pets to help control parasites and improve their nutrition:

Kittens: 1/2 teaspoon

Cats: 1 teaspoon

Dogs under 50 lbs.: 2 teaspoons

Dogs over 50 lbs.: 1 tablespoon

Dogs over 100 lbs.: 2 tablespoons

Cattle: 2% by weight of dry ration

Calves: 4 grams in morning

Dairy cattle: 2% by weight of dry ration

Chickens: 5% in feed

Goats: 1% in grain

Hogs: 2% of weight in feed ration

Horses:1/2–1 cup in daily ration

Sheep: 1% in ground grain

When I added garlic and food-grade DE to horse feed, it kept down the flies and mosquitoes around those horses that got these supplements.

Do not overgraze pastures. Parasites and their larva can be found on four inches of forage closest to the ground. Animals on overgrazed pastures graze closer to the ground, and therefore pick up more larva. Mow your grass short, remove yard clutter, and bring some sunlight into shaded areas.

Here are a few more benefits of food-grade DE for your animals:

• Cattle need trace minerals that come from DE

• Increases herd appetite, health, and production

• Helps stimulate the basic metabolism

• Increases protein digestion

• Satisfies and stops dirt-licking and corral-gnawing

About the Author

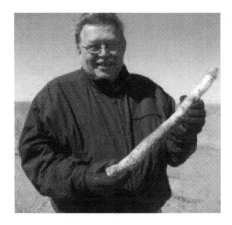

STEPHEN L. TVEDTEN was President of Stroz Services, Inc. (an alternative pest control company) for 25 years and President of Get Set, Inc., an integrated pest management company. He is President of PEST (Prevent Environmental Suicide Today), an environmental group, and founder of the Institute of Pest Management, Inc., Prescriptive Nutrients, Inc. and TIPM and the Natural Pest Control Association.

Steve is the consultant and advisor for Safe Solutions, Inc. and Head of the Advisory Board for the Natural Pest Control Council of America. Steve was licensed as a Michigan Residential Builder and Maintenance Alteration Contractor. He holds or has held pest control certifications issued by the states of Illinois, Indiana, Michigan, New York, Ohio, Texas, and Wisconsin.

CONNECT WITH STEPHEN TVEDTEN

To find out more information visit his website:
www.stephentvedten.com

BOOK DISCOUNTS AND SPECIAL DEALS

Sign up for free to get discounts and special deals
on our bestselling books at
www.TCKpublishing.com/bookdeals

Other Books by Stephen Tvedten

Natural Roach Pest Control: How To Get Rid Of Roaches Without Toxic Chemicals or Insecticides

How To Get Rid Of Lice and Nits Without Combing or Toxic Chemicals

Natural Bed Bug Treatment: How To Get Rid Of Bed Bugs Without Toxic Chemicals or Insecticides

Organic Spider Killer: How To Get Rid of Spiders Fast Without Any Pesticides, Chemicals or Toxic Poisons

How To Get Rid of Fleas: Kill Fleas Fast Without Any Pesticides, Chemicals or Poisons

Organic Ant Killer: How To Get Rid of Ants Without Pesticides, Toxic Chemicals or Insecticides

Natural Mosquito Control: How To Get Rid Of Mosquitos Fast Without Toxic Chemicals or Insecticides

One Last Thing...

Thanks for reading! If you enjoyed this book or found it useful I'd be very grateful if you'd post a short review on Amazon. Your support really does make a difference and I read all the reviews personally so I can get your feedback and make this book even better.

If you'd like to leave a review then all you need to do is click the review link on this book's page on Amazon here: http://amzn.to/13pszbk

Thanks again for your support!

Made in the USA
Las Vegas, NV
05 January 2024

83942508R00026